Instant Notes in Pathology

Instant Notes in Pathology

Dr.S.B.Asoka Dissanayake M.B.B.S (Ceylon)

Asokaplus

Asokaplus

Table of Contents

Chapter 01..15
    Introduction......................................15
        Approach to Pathology........15
        Learning Experience...........17
    Definitions..19
        Pathology............................19
        Disease................................19
        Pathogen 20
        Pathogenesis 20
        Pathogenicity 20
        Pathognomonic 21
        Pathophysiology 21
    How does pathology differ from other disciplines in Medicine?..........22
Chapter 02..29
    Approach to Para-clinical and Clinical Studies........................29
Chapter 03..31
    Basic Histological Features relevant to Pathology............................31
        Epithelial Cell Polarity........31
        Apical Differentiation.........31
        Cell Adhesion Molecules....32
        Cell Junctions.....................36

Chapter 04..41
    Acute Inflammation........................43
        Definition.............................43
        Agents of Acute Inflammation
       43
        Cells involved......................44
    Clinical features of acute
        Inflammation...........................45
    Steps in Acute Inflammation...........46
        Exudative Phase mainly of
            Plasma Fluids................46
        Cellular Phase......................46
        Homing in process involving
            Selectins and Integrins. 48
        Outcome / Sequelae 50
        Chemical Mediators............51
        Clinical Manifestations.......53
    Functions of Granulocyes................54
    Role of Liver in Injury and
        Inflammation...........................59
    Macrophage Functions....................60
        Primary Inflammatory
            Mediators......................63
        Differentiation in the
            Mononuclear Phagocyte
            System (MPS)...............65
        Monocytes...........................67

- Chapter 05..69
    - Chronic Inflammation......................69
        - Definition............................70
    - Classification of Chronic Inflammation...........................75
        - Chronic nonspecific inflammation................75
        - Granulomatous Inflammation. 76
        - Caseous Necrosis................77
        - Giant cells..........................77
        - Causes of Chronic Inflammation................78
        - Chronic inflammation due to other inflammatory cells 80
- Chapter 06..83
    - Cell Injury...83
    - 1. Free Radicals...............................84
        - Mechanism that generate free radicals..........................85
        - Mechanisms to clear Free Radicals........................86
    - 2. Chemical Cell Injury...................87
        - Cell Injury due to Alcohol...88
        - Toxic Effects of Ethanol......89

3. Cell Injury due to Impaired Energy Production...............................90
    Results of Decrease Energy Production....................91

Chapter 07...95
    Healing and Repair........................95
    Concept of Healing........................95
    Ability of cells for Regeneration or Repair..96
        1. Labile Cells....................97
        2. Stable Cells....................97
        3. Permanent Cells..............98
    Repair Process...............................98
    Healing of Skin...........................100
        Healing by primary intention 100
        Healing by secondary intention.....................100
    Factors influencing Wound Healing 101
    Pneumococcal Pneumonia............102
    Stages of bone healing..................103
    Growth Factors.............................104

Chapter 08...107
    Cellular Adaptation to Disease......107
    Hypertrophy.................................107
    Hyperplasia..................................108

Hypoplasia..................................108
Aplasia...108
Atrophy..109
Agenesis......................................109
Anlage...109
Atresia...110
Chapter 09..111
Immunology and Immunopathology
....111
Features of Immune System..........112
Cells of the Immune System.........117
    B Lymphocytes..................117
    T Cells...............................119
Antigen Presenting Cells...............122
    Cytokines..........................123
Classification of Immune Injury...129
Type I (immediate or anaphylactic)
    Hypersensitivity.....................129
Clinical Examples..........................131
Type II (antibody mediated cytotoxic)
    Hypersensitivity.....................132
Clinical Examples..........................133
Type III ((immune complex)
    Hypersensitivity.....................134
Clinical Examples..........................134
Type IV (cell mediated)
    Hypersensitivity.....................135

Delayed Type of Hypersensitivity (CD4 Cells)..........................135
Cell Mediated Cytotoxicity (CD-8 Cells)................136
Clinical Examples..........................137
Autoimmunity................................138
   1. Specificity.......................138
   2. Diversity.........................139
   3. Memory..........................140
   4. Self and Non-Self Recognition..................141
   5. Self Control or the Autoregulation............142
Organ Specific Autoimmune diseases 147
   Graves Disease...................147
   Hashimoto's diease............147
   Pernicious Anaemia...........148
Autoimmunity affecting Multiple organs and Tissues..................149
   Systemic Lupus Erythematosus (SLE). 149
Immunodeficiencies......................150
   1. Both B cell and T cell defects (SCID)............150
B Cell Defects...............................152

T Cell defects..............................153
AIDS..156
Human Immunodeficiency Virus...156
Chapter 10....................................161
Learning Outcome of Cell Death...161
Programmed Cell Death,
Apoptosis, Autophagy
and Necrosis................161
Apoptosis......................................162
Comparison and Contrast of
Necrosis and Apoptosis
......................................164
Necrosis..166
Coagulative Necrosis.........167
Colliquative-Liquefactive
Necrosis.......................168
Caseous Necrosis...............169
Gangrenous Necrosis.........169
Fibrinoid Necrosis..............170
Fat Necrosis.......................171
Autophagy....................................172
Chapter 11....................................175
Pigmentation.................................175
Accumulation of Exogenous
Pigments.................................175
Carbon in the lung.............175

Accumulation of Endogenous
　　　　Pigments...................................176
　　　　　　1. Melanin........................176
　　　　　　Hyperpigmentation............176
　　　　　　Hypopigmentation.............177
　　　　　　2. Bilibubin.......................177
　　　　　　3. Haemosiderin................178
　　　　　　4. Lipofuscin.....................179
　　　　　　Brown Atrophy..................180
Chapter 12...181
　　　Heterotopic Calcification..............181
　　　　　Dystrophic calcification....182
　　　　　Metastatic Calcification....183
Chapter 13...185
　　　Amyloidosis..................................185
　　　　　Amyloid............................185
　　　Other Physiological properties......188
　　　Classification of Amyloidosis.......189
　　　　　Primary Amyloidosis.........189
　　　　　Secondary amyloidosis
　　　　　(reactive systemic
　　　　　amyloidosis)...............190
　　　　　Other forms of Amyloidosis
　　　　　...................................191
Chapter 14...193
　　　Pathobiology of Disease................193
Fate of TB Lesion..203

        Atypical Tuberculosis...................206
Student Objectives....................................209
        1. Introduction..............................209
        2. Concept of Injury......................209
        3. Acute Inflammation..................209
        4. Chronic Inflammation...............211
        5. Cell Injury..................................212
        6. Necrosis and Apoptosis.............212
        7. Healing and repair.....................213
        8. Immunopathology.....................213
        9. Cell Adaptation.........................213
        10. Genetics and Disease..............214
        11. Calcification...........................214
        12. Pigmentation..........................214
        13. Amyloidosis............................215
        14. Metaplasia and Dysplasia........215
        15. Neoplasia................................215
        16. Disorders of Circulation...........216
        17. Cardiovascular System............217
        Authors Note.................................221

14

Chapter 01

Introduction

Approach to Pathology

1. Open Inquiry with Open Mind
2. Careful Observation
3. Logical and Critical analysis
4. Systematic Approach

    Six Levels

    1. At the level of whole organism

    2. System Level

    3. Organ Level

    4. Tissue Level

    5 Cellular Level

    6. Nano (Molecular) Level

a) Macroscopic Appearances

c) Microscopic Appearances

5. Ability gather information

6. Review and Revise Opinion or Judgment

7. Liberal Approach in thinking and assimilation of facts not personal beliefs

Discuss with peers

8. Take the given context as a Clinical Problem Improve one's Problem Solving ability and capacity.

9. Change or revise one's approach to a given problem to suit the needs of the given context. Do not be rigid and approach each problem as a new case not predetermined by previous experience and without prejudice.

10. Look for compromise rather than a rigid compartmentalized framework. When looking at a problem or when making Diagnosis

Learning Experience

Means of gaining new skills or improving the skills one already has like building a brick wall brick by brick.

Cognition

To know Pathology

Prior Knowledge of histology and physiology is essential.

New Knowledge is built on their foundation.

Construct an interpretation on a given problem.

Memory

Memory (rote memory) is not an essential part in learning pathology. What is necessary is to grasp the key concepts and their rational use in a given clinical problem.

Attitude

Open mind and open inquiry without prejudice.

Creativity

Essential core ingredient.

Power of Processing Clinical Data

Construct relatively a new way of

Thinking,

Feeling,

Doing

It is a continuous process

Not an end all or be all situation.

Definitions

Pathology

The study of structural and functional manifestation of disease.

Disease

Deviation from normal function or structure of any part of the
- Body, Organ or System

Manifested by
- Symptoms and
- Signs.
- Whose aetiology

(scientific classification causes of disease)
- Pathology
- Prognosis is known or unknown

Pathology is a branch of medicine studying basic or essential nature of disease especially in relation to changes in tissues and organs.

Pathogen

Disease causing microbial agent.

Pathogenesis

Development or evolution of a disease.

Pathogenicity

Ability to produce disease.

Pathognomonic

Characteristic feature depicting the pathology of a particular disease.

Pathophysiology

Altered state of physiology in a disease state, for example diabetes mellitus.

How does pathology differ from other disciplines in Medicine?

Even though, pathology is fundamental to learning of all the branches of medicine or surgery, it does not bear rigid compartments within itself except for organization and classification.

It deals with basic concepts underlying all the disciplines in medicine with appropriate integration to serve problem solving capacity in each field of study.

Even though, it does not inherit its own rigid compartment within a closed system, it can merge with any specialized discipline by way of basic concepts and these concepts can stand on their own theoretical base.

The attempt of this book is to identify those basic or core concepts and present them in a simple way with appropriate examples from a given system or branch or discipline.

Some examples may stand on their own and some concepts may fit within a given system but may not be readily discernible in another system. This does not mean there is some basic error of judgment in formulating the concepts.

It only means that the concepts are evolving systems and with more and more data crunching the ideal context or concepts change or refined.

One simple example is the response of the body to bacterial and viral infection.

The concept of infection is a concept within a basic concept called inflammation. The concept inflammation is somewhat rigid but the concept of infection is broad.

Within that broad concept of infection viral infections and bacterial infections behave in very dissimilar fashion.

The pathological study tries to compare and contrast the given scenario.

That is why when assessing pathology compare and contrast is a common question.

Similarly, genetic basis is a determinant of disease, but there may be a clinical problem that simulate a genetic preponderance but one cannot pin point a given gene or combination of genes to address the issue. Similarly there may be some masking effect by environmental or unknown factors. That does not mean that we throw away the concepts of genes and inheritance.

The other important approach in pathology is to open investigation and keep all avenues of investigation open at all times until one gets to the bottom of the problem like a forensic pathologist investigating a murder victim.

All the boundaries of a given problem is visited and revisited until a plausible explanation is provided and the scenario is mapped out in a given context.

This does not mean we find answers all the time, and it is just the opposite and at times pathologist may find the answers in about 60% of the time, at its best.

That is why pathology is interesting and challenging.

Coming from the old school of learning and teaching where student teacher relationship was considered very important and the student has to take part in active learning rather than passive assimilation of knowledge often not relevant to clinical demands writing another medical book may be redundant but careful afterthought decided to name it Instant Notes rather than concise notes.

This is a collection of instant notes I dish out often to their cell phones with core knowledge and concepts without filling or burdening their cell phone´s memory.

There were no illustrations and all were in PDF format.

Taking consideration of environmental foot print that paper based books entail and tablets and androids coming cheap this book is mainly for digital consumption.

However a limited paper edition will be available.

Chapter 02

Approach to Para-clinical and Clinical Studies

1. Aetiology

2. Definitions and classification of disease

3. Pathogenesis

4. Pathology

6. Microbiology

7. Immunology

8. Clinical Findings

9. Laboratory Findings

10. Differential diagnosis

11. Treatment Modalities

12. Complications

13. Prognosis

14. Prevention

15. Research

Chapter 03

Basic Histological Features relevant to Pathology

Epithelial Cell Polarity

Epithelial cells have major domains.
1. An Apical Domain
Protective (cilia in respiratory Epithelium) or absorption (microvilli in intestinal epithelium) or secretory properties
2. Basolateral Domain

Apical Differentiation

1. Cilia
2. Microvilli
3. Stereocilia

Cell Adhesion Molecules

A sheet of epithelial cells result from the tight attachment of similar cells to each other and to the underlying basal lamina (component of the extracellular matrix).

There are four major classes, two of which are Ca^{2+} dependent two which are not.

Calcium Dependent

1. Cadherins

Function as cell cell adhesion and morphogenesis.

Binds to actin through intermediate molecules called catenin.

E-Cadherins-Epithelial Cadherins

Homophilic (like and like) dimers

Trans homophilic (across two cells)

Heterophilic (like and unlike across two cells)

N-Cadherin

Central Nervous system, lens of the eye, skeletal and cardiac muscles

P-Cadherin

Placenta

2. Selectins

Each selectin has a carbohydrate recognition domain (CBD) with binding affinity to a specific oligosaccharide attached to a protein (glycoprotein) or a lipid (glycolipid).

Selectins participate in movement and localization of circulating neutrophils, monocytes and lymphocytes (leukocytes) to the tissues by a process called homing in or emigration.

P-Selectin

Found in platelets and activated endothelial cells.

E-Selectin

Found in activated endothelial cells.

L-Selectin

Found in leukocytes.

P-selectin is stored in cytoplasmic vesicles in endothelial cells. When endothelial cells are activated by inflammatory signaling, P-selectin appears on the cell surface.

Leukocytes have corresponding sialyl Lewis X antigen, a specific oligosaccharide which act as a ligand for P-selectin.

P-selectin binding slows down streaming leukocyte in blood and they begin to roll along the endothelial cell surface.

Calcium Independent

3. Immunoglobin Superfamily

N-CAM

Neural Cell adhesion molecule belong to immunoglobin superfamily and mediate homophilic and heterophilic interactions.

Adhesion molecules are coded by a single gene.

Members of the Ig family are generated by alternative messenger RNA splicing and have differences in glycosylation.

CD 4 and CD8 are members of the immunoglobin (Ig) superfamily.

These HLA antigens have variable immunoglobin like extracellular domains.

CD 4 Binds to Human Immunodeficiency Virus (HIV1).

Cell Junctions

Although cell adhesion molecules are responsible for cell cell adhesion, cell junctions are necessary for providing strength and stability.

Cell junctions are symmetrical structures formed between two adjacent cells.

There are three major classes of symmetrical cell junctions.

1. Tight Junctions

Tight junctions are called occluding junctions.

They have two major functions.

a) They determine epithelial cell polarity by separating the apical domain from the basolateral domains and preventing free diffusion of lipids and protein between them.

b) They prevent (paracellular pathway barrier) free passage of substances across an epithelial cell layer.

They have a belt like distribution and formed by occludin, claudin, nectins and junctional adhesion molecules (JAK).

2. Anchoring Junctions

Anchoring junctions are found below tight junctions and consist of three classes.

1. Belt desmosomes- Zonula adherence

They are associated with actin microfilaments through Cadherins.

2. Spot Desmosomes - Zonula Macula

They are associated with keratin intermediate filaments (also called tonofilaments) and extend from the spot to the lateral and basal cell surfaces of the epithelial cell.

They provide strength and rigidity of the cell layer.

3. The Hemidesmosomes

Consist of inner cytoplasmic plate associated with keratin intermediate filaments and outer membrane plaque linking the hemidesmosomes to the basal lamina by anchoring filaments composed of laminin and integrin.

3. GAP Junctions

The GAP junctions are not anchoring junctions but instead are communicating junction between two adjacent cells.

They are formed of integral membrane proteins called connexins.

4. Integrins

Heterodimers formed by association of alpha and beta subunits, encoded by different genes.

Intracellular domain binds to actin.

The extracellular domain binds to tripeptide RGD (Arginine, Glycine, Aspartate) sequence present in laminin and fibronectin two major components of basement membrane.

The integrin-extracellular matrix interactions are critical in cell migration to precise site in embryogenesis, homing in of cells to tissues and in sites of inflammation.

Intergrins responds to intracellular events by changing their extracellular adhesive conformations.

This is called ***inside out signaling.***

They form hollow cylindrical structures that span the plasma membrane.

Chapter 04

Learning Outcome of Acute Inflammation

1. Knowledge base
    - Starlings Principles of Fluid Movement
    - Change in Acute Inflammation
2. Outcomes
3. Sequence and complications
4. Causes and examples
5. Break down into
    - Vascular events
    - Cellular events
6. Vascular events
    - Vasoconstriction
    - Vasodilatation or Congestion
7. Cellular Events
    - Margination or Pavementation
    - Rolling
    - Adhesion

    Emigration

    Chemotaxis

8. Cells Involved

9. Time scale of events

10. The components Exudate vs Transudate

11. Chemical Mediators

12. Systemic Effects and involvement of the Liver

13. Acute Phase Reactants ACP

14. Benefits and Harm

15. Why Phagocytosis?

16. Bacterial Killing Mechanisms

17. Interaction with other Systems involved (Kinin, Coagulation and Complement System).

Acute Inflammation

Definition

Response of Vascular Tissue to Injury.

Agents of Acute Inflammation

1. Trauma

2. Physical Burns

3. Chemical Burns

4. Radiation

5. Injury due to abnormal Immune Responses

6. Infections

7. Sudden Loss of Blood supply (myocardial and cerebral infarction)-Ischaemia

8. Cell Necrosis.

Cells involved

Endothelial Cells

Polymorphonuclear Leukocytes

Neutrophils

Eosinophils

Basophils

Mononuclear Leukocytes

Monocytes and Macrophages

Lymphocytes and Plasma Cells

Tissue Resident Cells

Mast Cell

Clinical features of acute Inflammation

1. Pain (Dolor)

2. Redness (Rubor)

3. Swelling (Tumor)

4. Heat (Calor)

5. Loss of function (functio laesa)

Other characteristics

Sudden onset

Short duration

Leading cell is neutrophil

In addition

Systemic signs, fever and leucocytosis.

Steps in Acute Inflammation

Exudative Phase mainly of Plasma Fluids

Protein Rich Fluids

Cellular Phase

1. Intravascular Phase

Margination

Rolling

Adhesion

2. Emigration or Migration

3. Chemotaxis

      Unidirectional migration of cells

      ? over a Electro /Chemical gradient

4. Activation
- Arachidonic Acid Metabolites
- Secretion of Lysosomal Enzymes
- Respiratory Burst

5. Phagocytosis
- Bacterial Killing
- Removal or Demolition of Tissue debris

6. Bacterial Killing

Oxygen dependent Mechanisms
- Hydrogen Peroxide
- Hydroxyl Radical
- Hypochlorous acid

Oxygen Independent Mechanisms

    Lysozymes

    Hydrolases

    BPI (Bacteria Permeability Increasing Proteins)

    Defensins

Homing in process involving Selectins and Integrins

Leukocytes in circulation resit the shear forces to slow down along the vascular endothelium.

1. Rolling

Under condition of slow flow neutrophils / leukocytes make loose adhesion to endothelium and begin to roll.

Selectin in endothelial cells binds to carbohydrate ligands.

2. Adhesion

Chemical mediators in a site of inflammation stimulate the leukocyte to produce integrin beta 1 and beta 2 (Lymphocyte function antigen-LFA) on their surfaces. These ligands in turn bind to ICAM and VCAM receptors on endothelial cells.

TNF and IL1 produced by macrophages stimulate integrin production.

Integrin binding is firmer compared to selectins.

3. Transendothelial Migration
Emigration

This is also regulated by integrins.

This migration is facilitated by disrupting, the interaction of endothelial adhesion molecules to each other by leukocytes. The adhesion molecules disrupted are Junctional

Adhesion Molecules (JAM) and Vacular Endothelial Cadherins (VE-Cadherin) of the endothelial cells.

Up regulating of the beta 1 integrin by leukocytes facilitate migration.

Outcome / Sequelae

1. Resolution
 In Peumococcal Pneumonia
2. Suppuration and Abscess Formation
Staphylococcal and Ecoli infections
3. Scarring and Fibrosis due to tissue loss
Burns, Ulceration, Abscess
4. Leads to Chronic Inflammation (if not resolved).

Chemical Mediators

Gram Negative Infections
1. LPS
2. TNF
3. IL 1
4. IL 6 / IL 8

No PAF

Mediator Response

Vascular Dilatation

NO

Prostacyclin

Vascular Permeability

Histamine

C 3 a and C5 a

Bradykinin

PAF

Leukotries

Chemotaxis

C5 a

Leukotrine byproducts

Bacterial Particles

Interleukins and Chemokines

Clinical Manifestations

Fever

    IL1, IL6, TNF

    Prostaflandins

Pain

    Bradykinin

    Prostaglandin

Tissue Injury

    NO

    ROI (Reactive Oxygen Intermediates)

    Toxic Oxygen Radical

Functions of Granulocyes

1. Effector Cell in Acute Inflammation
2. Phagocytosis
3. Chemotaxis
4. Has receptors for Fc portion of immunoglobulin and complement C3b
5. Bacterial Killing

    Respiratory Burst-Oxygen Dependent Bacterial Killing

    Degranulation- Oxygen Independent Enzyme Activity

Acute Inflammation

1. Chemotaxis
2. Margination
3. Adhesion
4. Rolling

5. Emigration

7. Activation

6. Phagocytosis

>Helped by non specific opsonins

>Specific Immunogobins

>Fibrinonectin

>Fibrin

7. Bacterial Killing

>Degranulation

>Respiratory Burst

Stages of Development

1. Myeloblast

    Blue Cytoplasm

    Have Nucleoli

    No Granules

2. Promyelocyte

    Primary Granules

    Azurophilic granules

    Primary granules contain lytic enzymes, Elastases, Collagenases, Glycosidases

    Has Myeloperoxidase

    Acid Hydrolases

    Acid Phosphatases

    Cathepsins

    Lysozymes

    Phospholipase A2

3. Myelocyte

No nucleoli

Cytoplasm changes from blue to pink

Specific Secondary Granules appear and secondary granules gradually disappear.

Lysozyme

Phospholipase A2

Alkaline Phosphatase

Collagenases against Type II collagen

Cationic Proteins   Lactoferrin

Vitamin B12 Binding Protein

(No Peroxidases and Acid Hydrolases)

Tertiary Granules

Gelatinases

Early stage produce Enzymes of Anaerobic Glycolytic Pathway

Later stages produce Oxidative Pentose phosphate Pathway

58

Respiratory Burst

Cathepsins

Neutral Proteins

Note:

Hepatocytes in the liver produce enzyme inhibitors that include alpha 1 antiproteases and alpha 1 antitrypsin. There are other plasma and tissue inhibitors of elastase, cathepsins and alpha 2 macroglobulin.

Role of Liver in Injury and Inflammation

The role of liver in injury and inflammation is often little underscored. The liver almost immediately responds by producing large array of proteins. They are collectively known as Acute Phase Proteins (ACP).

C-Reactive proteins is one of the many acute phase proteins that are secreted almost immediately after bacterial infections.

Macrophage Functions

1. Scavenger Cell

Involved in removing tissue debris, apopototic bodies e.g; Myocardial Infarction.

2. Antimicrobial Defense (Antibacterial and Antiviral Activity)

Phagocytosis

Has receptors for Fc part of immunoglobin and complement

Respiratory Burst

Reactive Oxygen Species (Superoxide anion, Oxygen radicals, H_2O_2.

Have neutral proteases (Plasminogen activator, collagenases, elastases, cathepsins)

Lysozymes

Lipoprotein Lipases

Acid Hydrolases

ACE- Angiotensin Converting Enzyme

(No myeloperoxidase but monocytes in blood may have this enzyme)

3. Immunological Regulatory Function

　　Has Class II MHC which T cell recognizes

Accessory Cell　　　Antigen Presentation
Regulatory Cell　　Produce various cytokines

4. Storage Function　Pigments including iron, Abnormal Glycogens, Mucopolysaccharides.

5. Repair and Healing Process

　　Produce various Growth Factors (F.G.F, P.G.D.F, T.G.F)

　　　　Produce Fibronectin

　　　　Stimulate Angiogenesis

6. Regulate Coagulation / Fibrinolytic Pathways

7. Regulate Complement Pathway

8. Stimulate Bone marrow and granulopoiesis

9. Secretary Function
    1. Enzymes
    2. Oxidents
    3. Cell Adhesion Molecule-Fibronectin
    4. Inflammatory Mediators
    5. Immunoregulatory Mediators
    6. Coagulation Factors
        V, VII, IX, X, I
    7. Receptors for Fc, Complement, LDL, Factor VII
    10. Antitumour Activity
    11. Tissue Damage   TNF

Primary Inflammatory Mediators

1. Lysosomal Enzymes
    Acid Hydrolases
    Neutral Hydrolases
2. Cationic Proteins
3. Phospholipase A2
4. Prostaglandins
5. Leukotrienes
6. Cytokines IL1, IL 6 and TNF
7. Plasminogen Activator / Inhibitor
8. Procoaglant Activation
9. Complement Activation
10. Oxygen Metabolites.

Name	Location
Adipose tissue macrophages	Adipose tissue
Monocyte	Bone Marrow/Blood
Kupffer cell	Liver
Sinus histiocytes	Lymph node
Alveolar macrophage	Lungs
Histiocyte	Tissue macrophage
Giant cells	Granulomas
Langerhans cell	Skin and Mucosa
Microglia	Central Nervous System
Hofbauer cell	Placenta
Intraglomerular mesangial cell	Kidney
Osteoclasts	Bone
Epithelioid cells	Granulomas
Macrophage lining sinusoids	Red pulp of Spleen
Peritoneal macrophages	Peritoneal cavity

Differentiation in the Mononuclear Phagocyte System (MPS)

Committed cells within the mononuclear phagocyte lineage progress through a series of defined morphologically distinct stages. A common myeloid progenitor shared with granulocytes giving rise to monoblasts, promonocytes and then monocytes which migrate into tissues.

The production of mononuclear phagocytes from progenitor cells is directed by colony stimulating (CSF) factors which is hierarchical and lineage restricted and in their actions.

They include macrophage colony-stimulating factor (CSF-1), granulocyte macrophage colony-stimulating factor

(GM-CSF) and fms-like tyrosine kinase 3 ligand (Flt3-ligand).

These growth factors instruct the common myeloid progenitor to adopt a macrophage lineage.

Natural mutations in the CSF-1 gene in mouse provided the evidence that CSF-1 is required for the production of a substantial subset of tissue macrophages in the mouse.

The cells of the MPS are produced from pluripotent progenitor cells in the bone marrow. These cells require combined stimulus from CSF-1 and factors including IL-1, IL-3, GM-CSF and interferon-gamma to produce colonies in semi-solid medium.

Monocytes

These are larger than neutrophils (leucocytes) and posses large central oval or indented nucleus with clumped chromatin. The abundant cytoplasm stains blue and contains many fine vacuoles, giving a ground glass appearance. Cytoplasm may contain granules. The monocyte precursers in the bone marrow (monoblasts and promonocytes) are difficult to distinguish from myeloblasts and monocytes.

Chapter 05

Chronic Inflammation

Learning Outcome

The key to understanding of chronic inflammation lies on the biology of macrophages and their potential to withstand any onslaught and their ability to recruit other mononuclear cells at the site of injury or invasion. It is probably the oldest cell in evolution, in phylogenetical sense. The equivalent cell in early invertebrates is haematocyte which act as the sole defensive agent to intruders and irritant material. The lymphocyte probably did not cohabit in the early stages of life on this planet and evolved on a much later date and time scale.

Definition

Definition of chronic inflammation is difficult but its description can be overwhelming.

I would rather like to describe it in chess game parlance instead and leave the descriptive part in abeyance.

It is a stalemate condition in which the body's response is either faulty or inadequate to overcome the injurious agent which has gotten a foothold not easy to dislodge, resulting in injury, inflammation and attempt at healing by fibrosis.

All these processes go hand in hand either simultaneously or in successive stages.

The key elements are ongoing injury, tissue destruction (with or without necrosis) and healing by fibrosis (with or without calcification) and the persistence of the injurious agent.

It's clinical presence is

1. Insidious (onset)
2. Duration is long (weeks to years)
3. Cells Involved are mononuclear cells
4. Systemic signs may include fever, weight loss and anaemia.

While macrophage remains the major contributory cell lymphocytic infiltration is disproportionate tending to be either lymphocyte predominance or lymphocyte depletion. Whether these responses are immunogenic or in fact an aberration of the competency of the immune system are contemporary issues probably determined by production of inflammatory mediators in excess of the need.

The cell population is kept almost at a constant level either by cell division or by recruitment of new cells from circulation.

The ability of these cells to outlive their normal life cycle by avoiding apoptosis (without changing the course and transforming into neoplastic cells) is also an issue that is not resolved (at an academic level).

It is like two opposing armies are locked horned at the battle front in defensive position with neither army willing to go on offensive or *Kamikaze* mission for a decisive outcome.

The outcome vary from mainly macrophage accumulation in atherosclerosis to lymphocytic preponderance in aberrant immunological reaction and syphilis to a sum combination of and admixture of these two mononuclear cell lines in various combinations. (best seen in tuberculosis and leprosy).

It is not completely exclusive of other cells and there could be eosinophils, mast cells and even neutrophils at a site of chronic inflammation but their short life cycle and rapid turnover make them less distinct in comparison to the long present mononuclear cells at a site of chronic inflammation.

The clinical outcome may depend largely on nutritional status, especially in children.

A children with marginal nutritional deficiency may become protein calorie deficient (PCM) following a bout of measles which make them lose their appetite and also immunodeficient and then soon acquire tuberculosis which manifest as the fulminant miliary tuberculosis from which they die.

In this condition there are metastatic miliary tubercles in all the viscera and the full blown granulomas are rarely seen.

The cachectic syndrome that develops in tuberculosis leads to wasting and is the result of the production of various cytokines.

Classification of Chronic Inflammation

Chronic inflammation may present with two patterns.

Chronic nonspecific inflammation

It is also called mononuclear cell infiltration characterized by presence of macrophages, lymphocytes and plasma cells associated with granulation tissue and proliferation of fibroblasts. The monocytes are recruited to the site by chemical mediators. Macrophages in turn produce cytokines that activate and attract lymphocytes. Activated lymphocytes in turn secret additional cytokines that stimulate both macrophages and T and B cells (plasma cells).

Granulomatous Inflammation.

This type of inflammation is characterized by granulomas, which are nodular infiltration of macrophages that often morphologically change to become epitheliod cells.

Granulomas are often surrounded by a rim of lymphocytes and may or may not contain giant cells.

The cytokines are believed to play a role in change of monocytes to macrophages to epitheloid cells to giant cells.

Caseous Necrosis

Yellow cheese like (macroscopically) necrosis is often seen in tuberculosis.

In syphilis, the rubbery necrosis is called gummatous necrosis (gumma).

In sarcoidosis caseous necrosis is absent.

Giant cells

1. Langhan giant cells

2. Touton giant cells

3. Aschoff giant cells containing asteroid bodies and concentric laminated calcified bodies (Schaumann bodies)

4. Foreign body giant cells. Giant cells are not a feature but can be seen in viral infections and in some tumours.

Causes of Chronic Inflammation

Granulomas can form under diverse settings.

With persistent T-cell responses to Mycobacterium tuberculosis in which T cell derived cytokines are responsible for chronic macrophage activation.

Tuberculosis is the prototype of a granulomatous disease caused by infection.

Granulomas may also develop in immune mediated inflammatory diseases, for example Crohn disease, which is an inflammatory bowel disease that causes granulomatous inflammation.

They are also seen in a disease of unknown etiology.

The best example is sarcoidosis.

Granulomas can develop in response to relatively inert foreign bodies (e.g., suture material or a splinter) and then, they are called foreign body granulomas.

Chronic inflammation due to other inflammatory cells

Eosinophils are characteristically found in inflammatory sites due to nematode (filariasis and worm infestations) infestations. It is due to the immune mediated (IgE) response to large organism that cannot be ingested by the macrophages.

They aretypically associated with allergic reactions. Their recruitment is driven by adhesion molecules similar to those used by neutrophils and by specific chemokines (e.g., eotaxin) derived from leukocytes and epithelial cells. Eosinophil granules contain major basic protein, a highly charged cationic protein that is toxic to parasites.

Mast cells are widely distributed in connective tissues, throughout the body, and they participate in both acute and chronic inflammatory responses.

In atopic persons (those prone to allergic reactions), mast cells are "armed" with IgE antibody specific for certain environmental antigens. When these antigens are subsequently encountered, the IgE-coated mast cells are triggered to release histamines and arachidonic acid metabolites that elicit the early vascular changes of acute inflammation.

IgE-armed mast cells are central players in allergic reactions, including anaphylactic shock.

Mast cells can also elaborate cytokines such as TNF and chemokines and may play a beneficial role in combating some infections.

The presence of neutrophils is the hallmark of acute inflammation but few chronic inflammation may continue to respond with infiltrate of neutrophils.

A good example is actinomycosis.

In chronic osteomyelitis due to persistent presence of necrotic bone material, acute inflammatory cells continue to infiltrate and dominate the site of chronic bone injury/infection.

They are generally described as "acute on chronic inflammation".

Chapter 06

Cell Injury

Learning Outcome

Understand the mechanisms of cell injury.

Cell Injury

Pathology is the study of disease and disease processes.

All pathological processes that produce disease result from cell injury.

Cell injury set in a response that may or may not cause disease, hence understanding how cells and their contents are injured is of major concern of pathologists.

The basic concept is that all cell injury results in damage to the cell membrane.

Cells can be damaged directly or indirectly.

Direct Cell Injury.
>Free radicals.

Indirect Cell Injury.
>Toxins.
>
>Decrease in energy production.

1. Free Radicals

These molecules have single unpaired electron in the outer orbital.

They are unstable, highly reactive and set in motion active catalytic molecules.

Causes direct damage to the cell membranes. The liver damage caused by carbon tetrachloride is the model for free radical injury.

Other agents include, superoxide and hydroxyl radical.

Mechanism that generate free radicals

1. Oxygen toxicity

Alveolar damage in adult respiratory distress syndrome.

Retinopathy (retrolental fibroplasia) of prematurity.

2. Ultraviolet light.

3. Ionizing radiation.

4. Drugs.

5. Re-perfusion injury

Mechanisms to clear Free Radicals

Intracellular Enzymes

    Superoxide dismutase

    Catalase

    Glutathion peroxidase

Endogenous and exogenous antioxidants

    Vitamin C

    Vitamin E

    Vitamin A

    Cysteine

    Glutathione

    Selenium

    Ceruloplasmin and Transferrin

2. Chemical Cell Injury

The liver damage caused by carbon tetrachloride is the model for chemical as well as free radical injury.

In this model carbon tetrachloride induce P-450 mixed function oxidases in Smooth Endoplasmic Reticulum (SER) to produce highly reactive free radical of CCL_3.

The free radical thus formed diffuses throughout the cell initiating lipid peroxidation of intracellular membranes.

This leads to widespread injury, which include disaggregation of ribosomes, decreased protein production and failure of production of apoprotein moiety of lipoproteins and accumulation of fat (fatty change) in the cells.

Plasma membrane damage causes cellular swelling and influx of calcium (free calcium is a cell poison) with mitochondrial damage and cell death.

Cell Injury due to Alcohol

Ethanol is a universal cell poison that is more relevant than CCL_4.

We do not have an enzyme to metabolize alcohol hence we use alternative enzyme pathways that are vital for cell metabolism.

Ethanol causes reversible as well as irreversible cell damage.

Toxic Effects of Ethanol

1. **Fatty Liver**

Fatty liver results from inhibition of fatty acid metabolism.

It induces lipid peroxidation and inhibition of synthesis of lipoproteins.

2. **Hepatitis**

Alcohol induced hepatitis results from acetaldehyde and free radical generation from the live microsomal ethanol oxidizing systems.

3. **Cirrhosis**

Cirrhosis results from repeated hepatocellular damage, cell necrosis, (regeneration) and fibrosis.

4. Biochemical Injury

    Ketoacidosis.

    Lactic acidosis

    Hyperuricaemia

    Hypoglycaemia

3. Cell Injury due to Impaired Energy Production

Hypoglycaemia

Hypoxia

1. Ischaemia

2. Anaemia

3. Carbon Monoxide Poisoning

4. Cardiac failure and shock

5. Poor oxygenation due to pulmonary disease

Results of Decrease Energy Production

Decreased ATP production.

Impaired functioning of membrane ion pumps

Abnormal intracellular ion concentration.

Excess water into cells.

Damage to cell organelles.

Early Stage

Hypoxic cell injury first affects the mitochondria with decreased oxidative phosphorylation and reduction of formation of ATP.

Failure of cell membrane pump.

Increased intracellular sodium and water and decrease in potassium. This causes cell swelling or hydropic change.

Swelling of the endoplasmic reticulum.

Swelling of mitochondria.

Disaggregation of ribosomes and failure of protein synthesis.

Stimulation of phosphofructokianase activity results in glycolysis, accumulation of lactate and decreased intracellular PH.

Accumulation of hydrogen ions causes reversible clumping of nuclear material.

Late Stage

Hypoxic cell injury eventually leads to membrane damage.

This leads to formation of *cell blebs* most likely due to dysfunction of cellular cytoskeleton.

The formation whorl like structures called *myelin figures,* probably from damaged membranes is also a feature.

Ultimately, it leads to *Cell Death.*

Reversible Cell Injury	Irreversible Cell Injury
Intact cell membrane	Cell membrane disrupted
Cell Swelling	Damaged cells release lysosomal enzymes
Mitochondrial swelling	Protein Digestion
Endoplasmic reticulum swelling	Loss of basophilia
Detachment of ribosomes and proteins from SER	Leakage of enzymes and proteins
Hydropic or Vacuolar degeneration,	Surface blebs
Decrease of energy production. Increase glycolysis, decreased PH	Dense bodies in mitochondria
Lipid deposition	Initiate inflammation
Clumping of nuclear chromatin	Nuclear damage
	Pyknosis, Karyorrhexis and Karyolysis
Recovery is possible or May lead to irreversible cell injury if sustained	Cell death No recovery

Chapter 07

Healing and Repair

Learning Outcome

Know the process involved in healing / repair of injured tissue.

Concept of Healing

1. Removal of inflammatory debris

2. Regeneration of cells

3. Repair of the damaged tissue

4. Restoration to normal

Ideally all the above should be satisfied and it is rarely the case.

However, it is built in the system of the organism and depends on the availability of stem cells and their function.

It is the belief that one cannot change the inbuilt mechanisms but recent studies of stem cells in vivo is changing the attitude of the medical fraternity.

This is an area where active research should be encouraged and unravel the mysteries that surround biological systems.

Ability of cells for Regeneration or Repair

Cells are classified according to their ability of replacement from stem cells when lost or injured.

1. Labile Cells

These cells divide continuously in life to replace lost cells.

They have regeneration capacity.

These cells include cells lining epithelial tissue (skin, gut and blood vessels) and bone marrow.

2. Stable Cells

These cells remain as a stable pool and divide only when there is need for them (after injury or loss).

They include liver cells, renal tubular cells, mesenchymal connective tissues elements, like smooth muscles, cartilage and bone.

3. Permanent Cells

These cells have been considered incapable of division.

They are neurons and cardiac muscle.

They are replaced by fibrous tissue or glial tissue, after injury or loss.

(The above concept is challenged by recent and ongoing stem cell studies).

Repair Process

Living organism try to replace lost tissue due to injury or inflammation by either regeneration or repair.

Regeneration is seen in lower animals, such as seen in the gecko who manages to repair its tail after a misadventure. Many lower animals even able to grow lost limbs.

This ability is lost in higher animals and is replaced by a second best mechanism called repair.

Repair usually follow three stages.

1. Removal of debris due to injury or inflammation (demolition)

2. Formation of granulation tissue.

Granulation tissue consists of newly formed and proliferating capillaries and new blood vessels associated with fibroblasts that are synthesizing collagen.

3. Collagen synthesis replaces the lost tissue with fibrous tissue.

Healing of Skin

Healing by primary intention

    Clean surgical incision

    Cut injury brought together

    Regeneration of epithelial tissue

    Little granulation tissue.

    Little fibrous tissue

Healing by secondary intention

    Large defect

    Large granulation tissue

    More fibrosis

    Contraction of the scar tissue

Factors influencing Wound Healing

Local Factors

    Blood supply

    Persistent Infection

    Foreign bodies and debris

Systemic Factors

    Nutrition (Vitamin C, Protein, Zn)

    Diabetes mellitus (Infection, Vascular insufficiency)

    Steroids

    Anaemia

Pneumococcal Pneumonia

This is the typical example which illustrates the process called resolution.

Pneumonia leads to four processes that ends up in complete resolution.

1. Congestion

2. Red hepatization

3. Gray hepatization

4. Resolution

Stages of bone healing

    1. Haematoma formation

    2. Traumatic inflammation

    3. Demolition

    4. Formation of Granulation Tissue

    5. Woven bone and cartilage formation

    6. Formation of lamellar bone

    7. Remodeling

Growth Factors

There are many growth factors and few growth inhibiting factors. Their importance underlie not only healing but also transformation into malignancy (when somatic genetic mutations alter their behaviour causing them to multiply relentlessly and cause neoplasms).

1. Cytokines

    Interleukin 2 -T Cell Growth Factor

2. Colony Stimulating Factors

    Erythropoietin

    CSF

3. Macrophage Growth Factors

    IL1 and TNF

4. Growth of various Cell Types

1. Platelet Derived Growth Factor (PDEF)

2. Epidermal Growth Factor

3. Fibroblast Growth Factor

4. Transforming Growth Factor alpha (similar to EGF)

5. Insulin growth factor

5. Growth Inhibitors

Interferon gamma

TGF beta

Nitric Oxide

Heparan sulfate

Chapter 08

Cellular Adaptation to Disease

Learning Outcome

Understand and know the meaning of the terms Hyperplasia, Hypertrophy, Atrophy.

Hypertrophy

Hypertrophy is an increase of size of an organ or tissue by an increase in the size of the cells. Hypertrophy usually occurs in tissue composed of permanent cells (non dividing) such as skeletal muscle, cardiac muscle and smooth muscle.

Hyperplasia

Hyperplasia is an increase of size of an organ or tissue by an increase in the number of cells.

Hypoplasia

Hypoplasia is decrease in size of an organ usually due to developmental abnormality that produce decrease in number of cells. Hypoplastic organ tend to be normal in structure but small in size.

Aplasia

Aplasia is complete failure of development of an organ. The term aplasia is used when there is complete failure of cell regeneration in the bone marrow.

Atrophy

A reversible decrease in size of an organ or tissue due to decrease in size of the preexisting cells and not due to decrease in number of cells.

Atrophy may be physiological or pathological process.

Agenesis

Complete failure of organ to develop.

In contrast to aplasia no analge is present.

Anlage

Presence of primitive mass of cells.

Atresia

Hypoplasia or aplasia of a segment of a tubular structure such as blood vessels, bile duct, oesophagus and the intestine.

Chapter 09

Immunology and Immunopathology

Learning Outcome

Understand the concept of innate and adaptive immune responses.

Know the cell types and tissues involved in the immune system.

Be aware of causes and effects of immunodeficiency.

Understand the risk factors and pathogenesis of AIDS.

Understand the hypersensitivity reactions and their consequences.

Be aware of concept of autoimmune diseases.

Features of Immune System

1. Lymph nodes filter and screen lymph flowing from body tissues.

2. Spleen filter the blood.

3. T cell areas and B cell areas are separate in the lymph nodes and in the spleen.

4. B cells localize in the lymph node cortex as primary nodules which become secondary follicles with germinal centers, after antigen stimulation.

5. In the germinal centers, mesh work of *follicular dendrite cells* form from clonal expansion of B cell blasts.

They differentiate into *memory cells* and *plasma cells.*

6. Bone marrow is the major site of antibody production. Bone marrow start slowly

but produce long lasting production of antibodies.

7. The peripheral lymphoid tissue responds to antigen but only for a relatively short time.

8. Antigens and lymphocytes enter the spleen from blood stream through vascular sinuses.

Spleen lacks afferent and efferent lymphatics.

9. Lymphocyte recirculation between blood and lymph tissue is guided by specialized homing receptors on the surface of the High Walled Endothelium (HEV) of the post capillary venules.

10. High endothelial vessels are abundant in T-Cell zones of the para-cortex.

11. Macrophages are general antigen presenting cells for primed lymphocytes but cannot stimulate naive T-Cells.

12. **Dendritic cells** which process antigen migrate to the draining lymph node and settle down as interdigitating dendritic cells which initiate primary T-Cell responses.

13. **Follicular dendritic cells** in germinal centers bind immune complexes to their surface through IgG and C3b receptors. These complexes are long lived and provide a source of antigen stimulating for B-Cells

14. The medulla contain scattered lymphocyte, large number of macrophages and dendritic cells and in the draining site of immunization numerous plasma cells.

All of these cells are interposed between the lymphatic vessels / channels that drain the lymph node.

15. The activated plasmacytoid B-Cells migrate gradually from the follicular germinal centers to the medullary region of the lymph node.

This in effect prevent neutralization of antigen by high concentration of antibody in the follicular germinal centers.

16. The antibody produced are secreted into the lymphatic vessels.

17. MALT (Mucosa associated lymphoid tissue) or GALT (Gut associated lymphoid tissue) together with sub-epithelial concentration of cells lining the mucosal surfaces of the respiratory tract, gut and genito-urinary tract forms the *Secretary*

Immune System which baths the surface with protective IgA antibodies.

18. Special antigen transporting M-Cells provide the gateway for antigens that enter the mucosal lymphoid tissue.

Cells of the Immune System

B Lymphocytes

Cluster Domains

CD19   pan B cell marker

CD20   pan B cell marker

CD21   pan B cell marker receptor for EBV

CD22   pan B cell marker

Form plasma cells that secrete immunoglobins.

Has surface antigen receptors composed of immunoglobins.

B Lymphocyte Development

Pre-pre B cells   Rearrangement of heavy chain genes

Pre B cells   Cytoplasmic mu heavy chains

Immature B cells Surface IgM

Mature B cells   Surface IgM and IgD

plasma Cells   Cytoplasmic immunoglobins

T Cells

Cluster Domains

CD2 receptor for sheep red cells

CD3 attached to T cell receptor

CD4 helper T cells

CD5 pan T cell marker

CD7 pan T cell marker

CD8 cytotoxic T cells, binds to MHC class I antigens

Secrete lymphokines
Surface antigen receptor is attached to CD3
Rearrange gene for T cell receptor

T Lymphocyte Development

Prethymus stage

Surface markers TdT, CD34, CD38

Thymus Stage

Stage I surface markers CD2, CD5 and CD7

Stage II surface markers CD3, CD5, CD8, TCR

Stage III surface markers CD4 or CD 8

Postthymus stage

CD-4 positive helper T cells

CD-8 positive cytotoxic T cells.

T Cell Receptor

Analogous to B cell receptor (immunoglobins)

Composed of heterodimer linked to CD3

Binds to antigens attached to antigen presenting cells

Genes are rearranged only in T lymphocytes.

TCR-1

Composed of gamma and delta chains

Minority of lymphocytes.

Found in mucosal epithelium

Not associated with major histocompatibility complex

TCR-2

Composed of alpha and beta chains.

Majority of lymphocytes.

Associated with major histocompatibility complex.

Subpopulations

    CD-4 lymphocytes

    Helper T lymphocytes

    Respond to MHC class II antigens

    CD-8 lymphocytes.

    Cytotoxic T lymphocytes

    Respond to MHC class I antigens

Antigen Presenting Cells

1. Macrophages
    Phagocytic
    Produce cytokines
2. Dendritic cells in lymphocytes.
    Express surface HLA class II antigens
    Poorly phagocytic
3. Langherhan cells
    Found in epidermis
    Express surface HLA class II antigens

NK Cells

CD16 Receptor for Fc portion of IgG
    Large granular lymphocytes.
    Do not need previous sensitization.

Cytokines

Cytokines have many tropic actions.

They are pleotrophic (have many actions).

Actions last only nanoseconds.

Autocrine-Stimulate own cells

Paracrine-Stimulate cells in contact

Ecrine-Stimulate nearby cells

Endocrine actions when in excess.

IL-1

Secreted by macrophages, antigen presenting cells and other somatic cells.

Activate antigen presenting cells and helper T cells.

Stimulate neutrophils.

Stimulate B cells.

Induce fever.

Induce acute phase reactants.

IL-2

Secreted by T cells, macrophages and NK cells.

Stimulate T cell growth.

Stimulate helper T cells.

Stimulate cytotoxic T cells.

IL-3

Secreted by activate T cells.

Stimulate growth and differentiation of bone marrow.

IL-4

    Secreted by helper T cells.

    Stimulate B cell growth.

    Regulate heavy chain class switching.

IL-5

    Secreted by helper T cells.

    Stimulate and activate eosinophils.

    Stimulate B cell differentiation.

    Increase production of IgA.

IL-6

    Monocytes and T cells and other somatic cells.

    Inhibit growth of fibroblasts.

    Promote maturation of T and B cells

IL1, TNF and IL6 in high concentration induce shock.

IFN Gamma

Secreted by helper T cells, cytotoxic T cells and natural killer cells.

Potent activator of macrophages.

Stimulate neutrophils and NK cells.

Has antiviral activity.

Stimulate expression of class II antigens.

IFN alpha

Secreted by macrophages and B cells.

Has antiviral activity.

IFN beta

Secreted by fibroblasts.

Has antiviral activity.

TNF alpha - Tumour Necrosis Factor

Secreted by macrophages, T cells and NK cells.

1. Stimulate acute phase proteins

(Creactive proteins, alpha 1 antitrypsin, alpha 2 macroglobulin and haptoglobulin)

Prostagalndin E2 in hypothalamus.

Causes neutrophilia

2. Stimulate Endothelial cells

Increased leukocyte adherence.

Increased procoagulant effects.

Decreased anticoagulant effects.

3. Stimulate fibroblasts.

Increased fibroblast proliferation

TNF beta

Secreted by T cells.

Stimulate T cell proliferation.

Stimulate IL2.

Cytotoxic to tumour cells.

Classification of Immune Injury

Type I (immediate or anaphylactic) Hypersensitivity

First Exposure

Antigen binds to the antigen presenting cells.

T Helper cells secrete IL-4, IL-5 and IL-6.

B lymphocytes form plasma cells and produce IgE.

IgE binds to the Fc receptors of basophils and mast cells.

Subsequent Exposure

Degranulation

Antigen binds to the IgE bound mast cells and basophils resulting in degranulation of intracytoplasmic contents releasing histamine.

Secondary production of mediators

Mast cells and basophils synthesize new mediators which include arachidonic acid metabolites, platelet activation factor (PAF) and IL-4, IL-5 and TNF.

Eosinophilic infiltration

These chemotactic factors recruit eosinophils locally and also causes peripheral blood eosinophilia.

Clinical Examples

Atopic Eczema

Allergic Rhinitis

Hay fever

Allergic Asthma

Angioedema

Hives-Urticaria

Anaphylactic Shock

Type II (antibody mediated cytotoxic) Hypersensitivity

Complement reacting antibodies react directly with antigens.

The activation of complement system results in cytolysis.

Antibody dependent cell mediated cytotoxicity (ADCC).

The free Fc portion of the antibody react with the Fc receptor of various cytotoxic leukocytes, NK cells, monocytes, neutrophils and eosinophils.

Target cells are killed by Fc receptor bound cytotoxic cells and complement is not involved.

Clinical Examples

Haemolytic transfusion reactions

Autoimmune haemolytic anaemia

Rh incompatibility

Pemphigus vulgaris

Bullous pemphigoid

Graves Disease- Hyperfunction

Myasthenia gravis -Hypofunction

Pernicious anaemia -Hypofunction

Type III ((immune complex) Hypersensitivity

Formation of immune complexes.

Deposition of immune complexes

Complement activation and inflammation

Clinical Examples

Serum Sickness

Arthus reaction

Systemic Lupus Erythematosis

Polyarteritis Nodosa

Type IV (cell mediated) Hypersensitivity

Delayed Type of Hypersensitivity (CD4 Cells)

The T-Cell Receptor of the CD-4 cells interacts with antigens presented by macrophages and with HLA class II antigens on macrophages resulting in stimulation of specific CD-4+ memory cells.

On subsequent contact with the antigens the CD-4+ T cells proliferate and secrete cytokines.

IL2 and INF produce by CD-4+ cells recruit and stimulate macrophage and epitheliod cell formation and granuloma formation.

IL2 stimulate other CD-4 cells.

Gamma interferon stimulate macrophages.

Alpha interferon stimulate endothelial cells.

Cell Mediated Cytotoxicity (CD-8 Cells)

Cytotoxic T lymphocyte mediated cytotoxicity is the result of CD-8+ cells killing target cells directly. Typically virus infected cells and tumour cells are killed by this mechanism.

Specific target cell antigen is recognized by the T Cell Receptor of the CD-8+ lymphocytes. Target cell HLA class I antigens are also required for their activity.

Cytokines are not involved.

Clinical Examples

Tuberculosis   Mantoux Test

Leprosy   Lepromin Test

Granuloma formation

Contact Dermatitis

Autoimmunity

The fundamental mechanics of immunity can be rounded up in five rules.

If any one of them is violated that may lead to immune dysfunction.

1. Specificity

One antigen one antibody is the cardinal rule.

They are specific even to the nano level of molecular structure and are determined by antigenic determinant molecules. If the molecule does not have antigenic determinant that molecule will fail to activate immune cells.

This is very well seen in amyloidosis. The beta pleated structure of amyloid does not excite lymphocytes.

2. Diversity

Ability to respond to any antigen (within limits) is the second rule.

Variable regions in the heavy chains and light chains rearranges many a times in development of lymphocytes, giving rise to a vast array of molecules on the surface the lymphocytes, before and without exposure to antigens underlie the ability of the lymphocytes to respond to any given antigen molecule. These molecules on the surface of lymphocytes by random association find the best fit molecule (fit for purpose) for a given antigen molecule that brushes across them. Subsequent stimulation and molecular rearrangement at nano level makes the best available antibody to a given antigen.

If the molecule does not have an appropriate fit it will fail to excite the lymphocytes to produce antibodies.

Good example is seen in amyloidosis where beta pleated structure of amyloid proteins make them unavailable for immune response in spite of their protein backbone.

Not only lymphocytes, even macrophage cannot phagocyte them.

3. Memory

Memory of previous immune exposure is the rule that is not violated by immune competent cells.

Memory is fundamental to immune response. Once exposed and stimulated lymphoid system can recognize antigenic material almost permanently for life.

This is the economy of purpose, one does not have to reinvent the wheel, as it were.

4. Self and Non-Self Recognition

This rule again maintains the balance of self or non-self, foreign notion before mounting an immunological response.

In the early development of the lymphoid system any lymphocyte that may inadvertently react to a self antigen is carefully purged from the repertoire of naive lymphocytes.

5. Self Control or the Autoregulation

Any system that does not peter out, when no longer exists a need for sustenance, it is bound to fail in a biological system.

Good example of this failure is seen in a cancer cell.

A cell that becomes a cancer de novo and becomes autonomous and kills the subject as an end result illustrate this prophesy.

Immune system has checks and balances to prevent overshoot of its intended purpose.

In autoimmunity at least two of these rules are violated.

1. Inability to recognize self from non-self.

2. The other is the loss of self control.

In this context, the memory also becomes a handicap. The ability to produce diverse repertoire of antibodies makes the clinical response extensive and number of diseases produced far outweighs the immune system's responsibility to keeps homeostasis intact.

Why this has happened in evolution is a mystery.

Autoimmune responses are generally classified as organ specific or response of the other tissues to immune injury.

This classification is somewhat arbitrary.

Because of the response of the organ either by hyperfunction or by hypofunction one can easily detect the disease/s clinically but the underlying response/s of the immune cells do/does not vary a great deal, from their intended purpose in the normal immune response to foreign antigen/s.

In other words, if lack of clinical feature would blur what actually happens underneath, that does not mean that everything is hunky dory and fine under the hood at the cellular level.

Collagen diseases were coined for diseases of unknown aetiology. These encompass group of loosely related conditions most of which feature 'fibrinoid change" in connective tissue.

They may be autoimmune origin.

Antinuclear (ANA) and various other antibodies are found I collagen disorders.

Interestingly, fibrinoid material is frequently found in the placenta and why it occurs is ill defined.

I have my own explanation (based on my own research on placenta) for fibrinoid material in the placenta.

I treat it as an evolutionary bluff by the placenta to avoid foetal reaction to maternal antigens. This material collects in the foetal and maternal interface and the foetal Hofbauer cells (macrophages) are prevented from ingesting them as foreign material since the material in fibrinoid which include fibronectin act as a bluff and prevent mounting of massive immune response in the placenta. This material may be even coating the potential antigens preventing and exciting the immuno-competent cells in the placenta.

Similar mechanism may be at work when autoimmune components (antibodies) are coated with fibrinoid material and preventing further immunologically induced injury in the connective tissue.

This is an area one should do further research.

Organ Specific Autoimmune diseases

Hyperfunction

Graves Disease

    Thyroid stimulating autoantibodies

    Hyperthyroidism

    Exophthalmus

    Pretibial myoedema

Hypofunction

Hashimoto's diease

    Multiple autoantibodies

    Hypothyroidism

    Lymphocytic cell infiltration and Hurthle cell formation

Pernicious Anaemia

Auto-antibodies to parietal cells or intrinsic factor

Chronic atrophic gastritis

Vitamin B12 deficiency

Megaloblastic anaemia

Subacute combined degeneration of the spinal cord

Autoimmunity affecting Multiple organs and Tissues

Systemic Lupus Erythematosus (SLE)

SLE is a prototype of connective tissue disease.

Presence of ANA (antinuclear antibodies).

Extensive immune complex lesions.

Affect multiple organs system, joins, skin, serous membranes and especially kidneys.

2. Sjogren Syndrome

3. Polymyositis

4. Polyarteritis nodosa

Immunodeficiencies

1. Both B cell and T cell defects (SCID)

Marked deficiency in both T and B cells manifests as profound lymphopenia and deficiency in both humoral and cell mediated immunity.

X-linked form

Defect in IL2 receptor

Autoimmune Recessive form (Swiss Type)

Lack of adenine deaminase (ADA).

This enzyme deficiency leads to the accumulation of adenine triphosphate and deoxyadenine triphosphate both of which are toxic to the lymphocytes.

Associated with thymic hypoplasia.

Hypoplasia of tonsils and lymphoid tissue.

Severe infections.

Failure to thrive.

Malignancy

Graft versus host reaction.

B Cell Defects

X-Linked agammaglobulinaemia of Bruton

Defective maturation of B lymphocytes past pre-B cells due to mutation of the B cell tyrosine kianase.

Absence of germinal centers and plasma cells.

Bacterial infection begin after 6 months when maternal immunoglobulin protection weans.

Absence of immunoglobulins.

Common variable immunodeficiency

Variable clinical manifestation

Recurrent infections.

Hyperplastic B cell areas

Failure of terminal B cell maturation

Hypogammaglobulinaemia

Isolated deficiency of IgA

Usually asymptomatic

But may manifest as mucosal infections.

Recurrent upper respiratory tract infections

T Cell defects

De George Syndrome (Thymic aplasia)

    Developmental defects of the pharyngeal pouches 3 and 4

    Abnormal development of the thymus

    T cell defect

    Abnormal cell mediated immunity

Abnormal development of the parathyroid

    Hypocalcaemia

    Tetany

Typical facial appearance

    Wide set eyes (hypertelorism)

    Low set eats

Congenital defects of the heart and great vessels and recurrent infections.

It can be summed up by the popular acronym CATCH 22

    Cardiach defects

    Abnormal facies

    Thymic hypoplasia

Cleft palate

Hypocalcaemia

Microdeletion of chromosome **22**

Immunodeficiency with thrombocytopenia and Eczema (Wiskott Adrich Syndrome)

X-linked inheritance.

Characterized by eczems, thrombocytopenia and recurrent infections and poor antibody response to polysaccharide antigens.

Hyper IgM Syndrome

Both autosomal and X-linked inheritance. Normal level of IgM but failure of isotype switching to IgG, IgE and IgA. Increased incidence of pyogenic infections.

AIDS

Human Immunodeficiency Virus

Lentivirus, from Latin for lentis (slow) for slow progression of the disease.

Virion

Spherical envelope particle.

Diameter 100 nm.

Conical capsid with probable icosahedral symmetry.

Genome

Linear single stranded RNA, positive sense 9.3 kb.

Two identical genomes in each virion.

Cellular tRNA molecules packaged in virions used as primers for reverse transcriptase.

Genes and Proteins

Four capsid proteins.

Three enzymes Protease (PR), reverse transcriptase (RT) and integrase (IN).

Two envelope proteins.

Six regulatory proteins.

Viruses and Hosts

Human Immunodeficiency Types 1 and 2 (HIV-1 and HIV-2)

Simian Immunodeficiency Virus.

Equine, bovine and feline types.

Diseases

Acquired Immune Deficiency Syndrome

A major global pandemic with over 30 million infected.

HIV replicates in and kills lymphocytes and macrophages.

Infection results in depletion of CD-4 + cells rendering host immune deficient.

Opportunistic infection by other pathogens including avian tuberculosis may be fatal.

HIV-1 was probably transmitted to humans from chimpanzees infected with simian immunodeficiency virus.

Mechanism of HIV infection

The virus expresses cell surface protein gp120 with binding sites for the CD4 molecule on the surface of the CD-4 + T cells. In addition two two recognition sites on gp120 for the core-receptors CCR5 and CXCR4 are involved in viral entry into the cells.

Furthermore, monocytes, macrophages and dendritic cells are the target for viral infection and may act as reservoirs for HIV.

Pathogenesis of HIV

Depletion of CD-4 + cells and acquired immune deficiency.

Opportunistic infection by Pneumocystis jiroveci, Cytomegalavitus and typical and atypical mycobacteria such as Mycobacterium aviam intracellulare.

Chapter 10

Learning Outcome of Cell Death

Difference between necrosis, apoptosis, and degeneration.

Know different types of tissue necrosis.

Programmed Cell Death, Apoptosis, Autophagy and Necrosis

Programmed cell death is a very important concept without which the body will accumulate 2 tons of cells by the time one reaches 80 years of age.

Cell death is programmed.

It is genetically controlled.

Whereas necrosis is considered an accidental (non programmed) form of cell death in response to injury (acute hypoxic or ischaemic injury as a result of myocardial infarction).

Apoptosis

Apoptosis is derived from an ancient Greek word that suggests "leaves falling from a tree".

In contrast, to the swelling of the cell and its organelles that defines necrosis, the principle morphologic feature of apoptosis is shrinkage of the cell and its nucleus.

The distinction between apoptosis and necrosis is due part to differences in how the plasma cell membrane participate in these processes.

In necrosis early loss of integrity of the plasma cell membrane allows an influx of extracellular ions and fluid with resultant swelling of the cell and its organelles.

In apoptosis integrity of the cell membrane remains intact and persist until late in the process.

A key feature of apoptosis is cleavage of cytoskeletal proteins by aspartate specific proteases (capsase activation) which thereby collapses the subcellular components. Other feature include chromatin condensation (pyknosis), nuclear fragmentation (karyorrhexis) and formation of plasma membrane blebs and apoptotic bodies which are taken up by the macrophages.

There is no inflammation.

Comparison and Contrast of Necrosis and Apoptosis

	Coagulative Necrosis	Apoptosis
1. Stimuli or Injury	Hypoxia and Toxins	Physiologic/Pathologic
2. Histology	Cell Swelling	Cell Shrinkage
3. Nuclear Changes	Pyknosis, karyorrhexis and karyolysis	Chromatin condensation, Pyknosis / Fragmentation
4. Mechanism	Energy or ATP depletion	Events are energy dependent
5. Tissue Response	Cellular debris initiate Inflammation	Phagocytosis of apoptotic bodies by macrophages
6. Enzymes	Almost all enzymes from ruptured lysosomes	Endonucleases and proteases
7. Cell membrane	Disrupted at the beginning	Intact till late stages
8. Number of cells	Group of cells affected	Single or few cells
9. Progress	Disorderly	Orderly and programmed
10. Onset	Following Injury	Genetically determined

Examples Apoptosis

Embryogenesis and Organogenesis

Autophagocytic T cells in Thymus

Hormone dependent physiologic involution

In the endometrium during latter stages of menstrual cycle.

Chronic hepatitis C infection

Lack of apoptosis in malignant tumours

Tumour cell Death associated with chemotherapy and radiation.

Necrosis

Necrosis (from Greek neckrose for corpse) is best defined in the light microscope detection of cell swelling or rupture of surface membranes with spillage of intracellular contents.

The injury to cell membrane allows proteolytic enzymes to escape from lysosomes that initiate inflammatory response.

It is usually associated with rapid depletion of ATP.

The three nuclear changes that occur in necrosis are pyknosis, karyorrhexis and karyolysis.

The cytoplasm of a necrotic cell takes avid eosinophilic properties when stained with H and E staining.

Coagulative Necrosis

In coagulative necrosis dead cells lose their nuclei but the cytoplasmic outline of the dead cells remains intact.

This type of necrosis is called coagulative because the cytoplasm remains as a coagulated mass.

He "ghost" of these cells remain intact and the type of tissue can still be histologically determined.

It is also called structured necrosis.

Classic example of coagulative necrosis is myocardial infarction.

It is seen in solid organs like heart, liver and kidney.

Colliquative-Liquefactive Necrosis

Liquefactive necrosis differs from coagulative necrosis in that the tissue is totally digested and nothing remains, except the liquid component of the dead and inflammatory cells (called pus).

It is also called structureless necrosis.

In cerebral infarction (autolysis of dead cells) liquefactive necrosis is commonly seen.

Suppurative infections leads to formation of pus and colliquative necrosis.

Caseous Necrosis

Tuberculosis is the leading cause of caseous necrosis.

Macroscopically caseous necrosis has cheese like appearance.

On microscopic examination it is eosinophilic and structureless.

It consists of mostly coagulative necrosis but some liquefactive necrosis may also be seen.

Gangrenous Necrosis

This type of necrosis is seen due to vascular obstruction of the lower extremities and bowel.

Wet Gangrene

When complicated by bacterial infection and tissue digestion it is called wet gangrene. It is usually seen in untreated diabetes mellitus with vascular obstruction.

Dry Gangrene

When there is primary coagulative necrosis it is called dry gangrene.

Fibrinoid Necrosis

The appearance of fibrin like proteinous material in tissues and blood vessels is called fibrinoid necrosis.

It is also seen in rheumatic fever and in blood vessels in immune mediated vascular damage (polyarteritis nodosa).

Fat Necrosis

Results from trauma to fatty tissue (breast tissue) or due to enzymatic digestion of adipose tissue by pancreatic enzymes.

Autophagy

Autophagy which is derived from Greek "to eat" (phagy) oneself (self) was first used for structures that were observed on electron microscopy and that consisted of single or double cell membrane (lysosomal) derived vesicles containing cytoplasmic particles including organelles in various stages of disintegration.

It is a process by which cells recycle their own nonessential, redundant or damaged organelles and macromolecular components.

It is particularly prominent in cells undergoing atrophy induced by by nutritional or hormonal deprivation.

Note

Bulk protein degradation and organelle clearance occurs in two systems / pathways in eukaryotic cells.

The ubiquitin-proteosome pathway predominantly degrades short lived nuclear and cytoplasmic proteins.

The lysosomal-vacuolar pathway degrade larger substrate as protein complexes and organelles.

Chapter 11

Pigmentation

Pigmentation is classified into two broad groups.

When the pigments are products of the cell metabolism, it is called endogenous.

When the pigments come from food or exogenous material it is called exogenous.

Accumulation of Exogenous Pigments

Carbon in the lung.

Cinnabar in tattoo.

Lead in gingiva in lead poisoning.

Carotene from plant foods

Accumulation of Endogenous Pigments

1. Melanin

This pigment is formed from tyrosine by the action of tyrosinase and is synthesized in the melanosomes in melanocytes resident in the basal layer of the epidermis. Each melanocyte transfers its melanin synthesized to a cluster of 30 to 35 keratinocytes.

Macrophage also can take up melanin to its melanophores.

Hyperpigmentation

Increased melanin pigmentation associated with sun tanning and variety of disease conditions.

Hypopigmentation

Decreased melanin pigmentation associated with albinism and vitiligo.

2. Bilibubin

This pigment is the catabolic product of the haeme moiety of the haemoglobin and to a minor extent from myoglobin.

The increase in bilirubin produce jaundice which discolors the sclera, mucosa, blood vessels and internal organs.

It causes brown discoloration of the liver.

Causes

1. Haemolytic anaemia due to excessive haemolysis of red cells.

2. Hepatocellular jaundice due to parenchymal liver cell damage (hepatitis).

3. Obstructive jaundice due to intra and extra hepatic obstruction of the biliary ducts and canaliculi.

3. Haemosiderin

The iron containing pigment of aggregates of ferritin seen in macrophages and parenchymal cells (liver).

It appears in tissues as golden brown colour and stains blue with Prussian blue dye.

It accumulates pathologically in excess amounts in;

Haemosiderosis due to multiple blood transfusions in spherocytosis or thalasaemia.

Hereditary Haemachromatosis it accumulates in macrophages and parenchymal tissues.

It causes damage to liver, pancreas and testicles. The classic triad of skin pigmentation, diabetes mellitus and cirrhosis is called "Bonze Diabetes".

4. Lipofuscin

A fine granular golden brown fat soluble pigment within lysosomes as a result of lipid peroxidation of plasma membranes.

Lipofuscin is a "wear and tear pigment that is most commonly seen in hepatocytes and heart muscle of elderly individuals or patient with severe malnutrition.

Brown Atrophy

The combination of atrophy of organs and accumulation of lipofuscin is referred to as brown atrophy.

Chapter 12

Heterotopic Calcification

This is defined as the deposition of calcium salts I tissues other than osteoid, dentine or enamel. Because calcium salts are radio-opaque, their deposition is conspicuous on radiographs.

Microscopically calcium salts appear as granular deposits which stain dark blue with H and E.

Two distinct type of calcification are recognized.

Dystrophic calcification

Dystrophic calcification is the deposition of calcium in dead or degenerative tissue. The plasma levels of calcium and phosphate are normal and the abnormal local conditions are the cause of calcification.

Caseous material in tuberculosis.

Haematoma

Infarcts

Atheroma

Heart Valves

Meningioma

Cysts

Calcinosis in systemic sclerosis

Metastatic Calcification

Metastatic calcification is due to abnormality of calcium metabolism resulting in high levels of serum calcium. The calcification takes place in normal tissues including organs such as in kidneys (nephrocalcinosis) resulting in renal failure.

There are many causes of hypercalcaemia.

Hyperparathyroidism

Vitamin D toxicity

Sarcoidosis

Metastatic cancer of bone

Chapter 13

Amyloidosis

Amyloid

A fibrillary protein of heterogeneous origin that has the characteristic beta pleated sheet configuration (appearance) when viewed under x-ray diffraction crystallography.

It stains brown with iodine, pink with hematoxylin and eosin stain and dark red with congo red stain.

When viewed under polarized light, amyloid stained with congo red stain displays an apple-green birefringence.

Amyloid appear identical on light microscopy.

In H and E amyloid appear as hyaline, structureless and eosinophilic material.

It was thought to be a starch like substance due to its iodine staining.

The starch like component is minor component (10%) of amyloid. It consists of a globular pentagonal subunit (P component) having the chemical composition as normal alpha-1 serum glycoprotein, closely related to CRP (C-Reactive Protein).

Being a glycoprotein it is responsible for the variable positive staining with PAS. However, it does not contribute to the beta pleated structure of the longitudinal fibrils.

Amyloid consists of different fibrillary (non branching) proteins (90%) which are arranged in a common beta pleated structure. Each fibril is composed of two or more filamentous subunits orientated longitudinally.

Cross beta pleated configuration is the feature common to all amyloid.

Amyloid consists of three component.

1. Variable beta pleated component (90%).

2. Glycoprotein component (Amyloid P component-10%).

3. Minor components

GAG-(Glycosamineglycans)

PG(Proteoglycan)

Laminin, fibronectin, type IV collagen

Basement membranes

Other Physiological properties

It is non-toxic and inert.

It is not immunogenic.

It cannot be phagocytosed by macrophages.

It does not excite inflammation.

It is a physiochemically bland material.

It accumulates extracellarly. It accumulates in blood vessels. It impairs transfer of nutrients across blood vessels. It fills up among cells in the extravascular tissue and causes pressure atrophy and or ischaemic injury. Impair vascular homeostasis and coagulation. It impairs permeability of glomerular basement membranes causing proteinuria. It impairs function by interfering with contraction of the myocardium.

Classification of Amyloidosis

Classification of amyloidosis is somewhat arbitrary.

Primary Amyloidosis

Primary amyloidosis is the form usually associated with plasma cell dycrasias, such as multiple myeloma and Waldenstrom macroglogulinaemia.

Immunoglobulin light chain referred to as AL (amyloid light chain) protein or Bence John protein is seen in multiple myeloma

Amyloid deposition is usually mesodermal in distribution but may involve kidneys.

Secondary amyloidosis (reactive systemic amyloidosis)

Secondary amyloidosis is usually a complication of chronic inflammatory diseases, such as rheumatoid arthritis, tuberculosis, osteomyelitis, syphilis and leprosy.

The protein fibrils are formed from AA protein (amyloid associated) which is derived from SAA (serum amyloid associated protein).

SAA is actually an acute phase reactant produced in chronic inflammatory diseases.

Amyloid deposition is usually visceral in distribution (liver, spleen, pancreas).

Other forms of Amyloidosis

1. Senile amyloidosis

2. Insulin resistant diabetes mellitus

3. Medullary carcinoma of thyroid

4. Alzheimer's Disease

5. Familial Mediterranean Fever

6. Portuguese type of polyneuropathy

Chapter 14

Pathobiology of Disease

This is an introduction for students who commence their clinical work.

Pathological processes involved in *Chronic Inflammation* is illustrated as an example.

For example consider tuberculosis. Tuberculosis causes apical pneumonia which is a chronic infection in the lung. If spontaneous recovery does not follow tuberculosis leads to many complications.

The causative organism is mycobacterium (Mycobacterium tuberculosis).

Susceptible subjects are children under 5 years and adult over 45 years.

Contributory factors may be diabetes mellitus, alcoholism, immune deficiencies, poor nutrition, AIDS and people living in poor residential facilities.

The ***Primary Pathology*** *is the* **Chronic Inflammatory Response**.

Terminology used when the lung is affected is ***Apical Pneumonia***.

Usually results in destructive changes in the lung, for example ***Cavity Formation***.

Pleural effusion is a complication.

Metastatic spread of the infection leads to **meningitis** and generalized **miliary tuberculosis.**

Each of the *primary pathology, the secondary pathology* and *complications* produces its own *symptoms and signs*.

Microbiology

This illustrates the microbiological features.

Aetiology

Other Organisms involved are

Mycobacterium tuberculosis

Mycobacterium avium

Mycobacterium tuberculosis
Morphology

Slender bacillus

Non motile, non sporing

Staining

Ziel Neelson Method

Waxy wall is impermeable to Gram stain.

Takes up heated stain

Stain with Carbol Fuchsin stain

Counter stain with Methyl Blue or Malachite Green.

Resist decoloration by strong Acids and Alcohol (H_2SO_4, Absolute Alcohol)

Acid fast material is stained red.

Culture

Lowenstein Jenson Medium (Egg yolk, Glycerol)

Takes 6 to 8 weeks

Animal inoculation

Guinea pigs (poor fellows)

Other Features

Resistant to drying out but sensitive to sunlight and UV light.

Virulence

Vary according to the type of micro-organism and the host animal.

Antibiotic Sensitivity

    Multiple drug resistance

Other Pathological Lesions

    Miliary tuberculosis

    Meningitis

    Intestinal tuberculosis

Vaccination

    BCG

    Effectiveness is debated but safe enough with only local complications.

Clinical Symptoms and Signs

Incubation period

may be long with malaise.

Symptoms may include high fever, nocturnal sweating and wasting.

Signs of pneumonia and cavity formation in the lung

Fibrosis of tissues affected

Healing with fibrosis and calcification

End result may be chronic debilitating illness without treatment.

Pathology

Macroscopy	Microscopy
Caseation	Granuloma Formation
Coagulative Necrosis	
Caseation	
Mechanism of Injury	Hypersensitivity
	Delayed Type
Cellular Response	Monocytic
Chemical Mediators	TNF
	IL-1
	IL-2
	IL-6

Progress

Healing by fibrosis and calcification

Caseation with tissue destruction

Caseous, Fibrocaseous and Fibroid Lesions

Predisposing Factors

    Age below 5 years

    Old age

    Over 45 years

    Diabetes mellitus

    Protein malnutrition

    Immunodeficiency

    Following Measles

    AIDS

Pathogenesis of Tuberculous Lesion

1. Transient acute inflammatory reaction.

2. Infiltration of monocytes.

3. Macrophages phagocyte the bacilli but no actual killing.

The cytoplasm and nucleus change.

The cytoplasm pale and eosinophilic. The nuclei are elongated and vesicular.

They are called EPITHELOID cell

4. These epitheloid cells fuse to form Langhan's Giant cells.

5. Round cell infiltration with lymphocytes and plasma cells.

6. In 10 to 14 days central necrosis.

7. Healing by fibrosis

a. Proliferative cell reaction

b. Exudative reaction in serous cavities for example pleural effusions

Fate of TB Lesion

Hallmark of Healing

Healing by fibrosis, calcification, even ossification.

Hallmark of Activity

CAESATION

Softening and discharge of sputum and bacteria.

Spread

1. Local Spread

2. Lymphatic spread

3. Blood stream spread (military tuberculosis)

4. Serous Cavities (tuberculous meningitis.

5. Epithelial surfaces (tuberculous enteritis).

Childhood Tuberculosis

Childhood	*Adult*
1. Primary Focus (Ghon's focus) Sun-pleural focus heals	Apical / sub-apical Assmann Focus)
2. Local spread	
Massive enlargement of the Hilar nodes	Caseation
	Cavity formation
Caseation	Heals by fibrosis
Heals and calcify	Lymph node enlargement is inconspicuous
Blood stream spread	Blood stream spread is rare.
Miliary tuberculosis and meningitis	

Gastrointestinal tuberculosis

Primary focus is small.

Small primary focus and tendency for extensive lymph node enlargement.

Swallowed infected sputum.

Tuberculous peritonitis.

Ulceration of the ileum.

Extensive local destruction with little lymphatic involvement.

Extensive fibrosis and stricture formation.

Atypical Tuberculosis

Pathological manifestation are similar but clinical presentation is different.

Usually affect cervical glands in children.

Scrofula is the term used for lymphadenopathy of the neck, usually as a result of an infection in the lymph nodes, known as lymphadenitis.

It can be caused by tuberculous or non tuberculous mycobacteria.

The classical histological pattern of cervical lymphadenitis (scrofula) features caseating granulomas with central acellular necrosis (caseous necrosis) surrounded by granulomatous inflammation with multinucleated giant cells.

Although tuberculous and non tuberculous lymphadenitis are morphologically identical, the pattern is somewhat distinct from classical tuberculosis.

Scrofula is often caused by atypical mycobacteria (*Mycobacterium scrofulaceum*) and other non-tuberculous mycobacteria (NTM).

This classification was proposed by one of my teachers of microbiology after extensive local studies.

I can remember him getting a skin lesion in his face due to inoculation by one of these strains. He was smart enough to get it excised (the lesion) by a surgeon and cover it with a skin graft (without scars) with minimal tell tale signs.

Unfortunately, his work was not recognized due to some professional rivalry and he gave up microbiology and became a psychiatrist.

Before he migrated to Australia, I can remember him telling me, it is far better to become a psychiatric, so he could understand the mentality of the guys who read his colossal work and refuse to recommend it.

There was a rumble at that time, the real reason for rejecting the thesis (this was the first medical PhD thesis done locally at that time) was to prevent local work being published, so the guys and girls could go abroad for their PhDs and obtain the perks associated them.

This made me to rethink staying in Sri-Lanka and I followed him to UK.

It is not an exaggeration to say he was one of the brightest products of our university. He had five boys and all of them are holding good posts abroad currently.

Student Objectives

1. Introduction

Understand the meaning of the terms Pathology, aetiology, pathogenesis and Prognosis.

Understand different types of mechanisms which result in disease.

Know the different disciplines that make up the study of Pathology.

2. Concept of Injury

Know the agents of injury

Know the types of injury

Know the duration (short or long)

Know the effect of injury (recurrent or persistent)

Know the response of the living tissue

3. Acute Inflammation

Understand the process and purpose of inflammation.

Know the cardinal features of inflammation.

Nature and differences between acute and chronic inflammation.

Know the duration

Know the types of injury

Know clinical outcome

Know the cardinal signs

Know the vascular response

Know the cellular response

Know the role of neutrophil (phagocytosis and bacterial killing)

Know the role of macrophage (demolition and repair)

Know the role of lymphocytes (in acute bacterial infections)

Know the chemical mediators

Should be able compare and contrast exudate from transudate

Should be able explain the sequelae including resolution, demolition, abscess formation, repair, healing and final outcome.

4. Chronic Inflammation

Know the duration

Know the types of injurious agents

Know clinical outcome

Know the clinical signs

Know the cellular response

Know the role of macrophage (phagocytosis, bacterial killing, epitheliod cell formation, giant cell formation, necrosis and recruitment of other cells-lymphocytes)

Know the role of macrophage (demolition and repair)

Know the role of lymphocytes (in chronic bacterial infections)

Know the role chemical mediators

Know the type of tissue response

Should be able compare and contrast granulomatous and non-granulomatous lesions

Should be able explain the sequelae including demolition, repair, healing, fibrosis, calcification, recurrence of injury and final outcome.

Should know in detail

Tuberculosis

Leprosy

Syphilis

Sarcoidosis

Chronic osteomyelitis

Rheumatic Fever

5. Cell Injury

Understand the mechanisms of cell injury.

6. Necrosis and Apoptosis

Difference between necrosis, apoptosis, and degeneration.

Know different types of tissue necrosis.

7. Healing and repair

Know the process involved in healing / repair of injured tissue.

8. Immunopathology

Understand the concept of innate and adaptive immune responses.

Know the cell types and tissues involved in the immune system.

Be aware of causes and effects of immunodeficiency.

Understand the risk factors and pathogenesis of AIDS.

Understand the hypersensitivity reactions and their consequences.

Be aware of concept of autoimmune diseases.

9. Cell Adaptation

Understand and know the meaning of the terms Hyperplasia, Hypertrophy, Atrophy.

10. Genetics and Disease.

Know the normal human chromosome complement.

Understand chromosomal abnormalities with Down's syndrome as an example.

Be aware of different patterns of inheritance of single gene disorders.

Be aware of investigations of genetic disorder.

11. Calcification

Know the two types and the relationship to calcium metabolism.

Dystrophic

Metastatic

12. Pigmentation

Know the types and pigments involved.

Endogenous

Exogenous.

13. Amyloidosis

Know the properties of amyloid.

Know the staining properties.

Know the simple classification.

14. Metaplasia and Dysplasia.

Define metaplasia
Define dysplasia

15. Neoplasia

Understand the basic concept of oncogenesis, oncogenes.

Have the knowledge of treatment modalities available for malignant neoplasms.

Define term neoplasia, tumor, cancer, carcinoma and sarcoma.

Know the distinction between benign and malignant neoplasms.

Understand the basis of tumour classification, nomenclature.

Understand the concepts of tumor grade and stage.

16. Disorders of Circulation

Understand the meaning of Ischemia, infarction, thrombosis and embolism.

Know the risk factors for and understand the pathogenesis of atherosclerosis.

Understand the meaning of terms Oedema, shock and cardiac failure.

Systemic Pathology

17. Cardiovascular System

Understand Ischaemic heart disease, coronary heart disease.

Understand heart failure.

Mechanism and effects of Hypertension.

Valvular heart disease & Pathogenesis of Rheumatic fever (review)

Effects of Heart disease

18. Respiratory System

Respiratory tract infections, Pneumonia.

Asthma & Allergy.

Tuberculosis, pathogenesis and effects.

Lung Cancer, risk factors and pathogenesis.

19. Gastrointestinal System

Understand causes and management of Peptic Ulcer disease.

Understand digestion, disorders of Malabsorption.

Understand terms diarrhoea, constipation, causes and management.

Infections of GIT

Appendicitis and Typhoid

Understand the mechanisms of Intestinal Obstruction.

Tumors of intestine.

Cancer of colon.

20. Liver & Pancreas

Understand liver diseases, Jaundice, causes and management.

Alcoholic liver disease

Pathogenesis and complications

Viral Hepatitis

Understand complications & Routes of spread

Gall stones and their effects.

Pancreatitis - types & effects

21. Hematology

Diseases of blood and blood forming organs.

Understand the significance of common blood tests, "penias & philias"

Anemia

Understand and its causes and management

Understand White cells and their significance in diseases

Understand the term Leukemia major types, modality of treatment.

Understand Haemostasis, coagulation with example, Haemophilia

22. Urinary system

Understand common Disorders of Kidney, and their manifestation

Understand terms Nephritic syndrome, nephrotic sysndrome, Glomerulonephritis

Pyelonephritis

Chronic kidney disease,

End stage kidney.

Understand causes and management of Renal calculi.

Infections, tumors & obstruction of urinary tract.

23. Nervous System

Special features of nerve cells, and brain

Head injury, its effects, understand terms cerebral edema, hematoma

Understand Cerebral infarction, hemorrhage and their effects.

Infections types septic/aseptic, Understand meningitis & encephalitis.

Degenerations - Alzheimers disease.

Understand tumors of brain, their types and effects.

24. Miscellaneous

Sexually transmitted diseases

Reproductive system-cervical cancer, PAP smear.

Common diseases of male genital system - BPH, carcinoma prostate.

Arthritis, rheumatoid, osteoarthritis.

Osteomalacia and Osteoporosis.

Authors Note

In Part I, of this book I have left out three big chunks of information to be included in the Part II of the series.

They include,

1. Genetic basis of pathology

2. Vascular and circulatory disorders

3. Neoplasia

Reason for not including neoplasia is because of its importance and extensive information that need to be organized in a logical basis.

Equally, genetic factors and viral aetiology are interlinked with neoplastic transformation.

Reason for excluding cardiovascular pathology is obvious that it should be better organized under systemic pathology.

Asokaplus

www.ingramcontent.com/pod-product-compliance
Lightning Source LLC
Chambersburg PA
CBHW020901180526
45163CB00007B/2589